THE PALEO KID:

26 Easy Recipes
That Will Transform Your Family
(Primal Gluten Free Kids Cookbook)

Kate Evans Scott

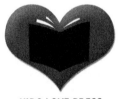

KIDS LOVE PRESS

This book is dedicated to my two beautiful children.

TABLE OF CONTENTS

BREAKFAST MENU

LUNCH MENU

DINNER MENU

DESSERT MENU

CONDIMENTS

ACKNOWLEDGMENTS

Thank You to all of my friends and family for your support and encouragement - your guidance has helped me bring this book to fruition. I could not have done it without you. I would also like to thank all of the wonderful food lovers out there who have given me so much inspiration over the years to eat healthier and enjoy doing it at the same time!

UH-OH, PALEO! WHAT IS THIS DIET?

Starting on the Paleo diet is like taking a step back in time... way back in time... It's a gastro-adventure that takes you backward two million years to the Paleolithic era, when humans were a hunter-gatherer society. That means that people lived on wild game and the plants, fruits and nuts they gathered from their environment.

When human beings started cultivating grains and raising animals for meat and dairy 10,000 years ago, we began suffering from chronic illnesses like heart disease, type 2 diabetes, obesity, depression, memory loss and other inflammatory diseases. Tribal people living today that eat similar diets to our Paleolithic ancestors do not suffer from these life-threatening diseases. We have to assume that it has to do with their diet and lifestyle.

If you do the Paleo diet right, you won't feel hungry and crave the foods you've eliminated. Instead, you'll feel satiated, vibrant and healthy!

WHAT DO WE EAT NOW?

While there is much debate about exactly what you can and can't eat on the Paleo diet, it's best for kids to start with a simple-to-follow framework for their eating habits. If you are trying to address very specific dietary needs, like food allergies or celiac, then of course you'll want to stay away from those foods. Also, people choosing Paleo as a weight loss program will want to stay away from starchy vegetables like potatoes, and refrain from eating too many dried and fresh fruits.

But since most children are very active- much like our running, jumping, hiding, walking, swimming Paleolithic ancestors- they shouldn't have to worry too much about starches and fats.

BASIC FOOD LIST

Here is a food guideline to get you started. Remember, there is a little bit of wiggle room, as even the Paleo diet experts disagree about certain foods. If you are unsure, you should always do your own research and tailor your diet to your specific needs.

Vegetables and Sea Vegetables: You can eat any and all vegetables. In fact, you should eat a "rainbow" of vegetables, from red to violet, in order to give your body a wide variety of vitamins and nutrients. Sea veggies, like seaweed and algae, are especially good for you.

Fruits: Eat all the fruits. These can be fresh, cooked, or dried. However, if you're trying to lose weight or if you have a problem with tooth decay, you may want to limit dried fruits.

Meats, Fish & Eggs: You will eat a lot of meat and eggs on the Paleo diet, as did our hunter-gatherer ancestors. Protein plays a huge role in proper brain and muscle development, and since you're not going to eat any legumes or grains, meat and eggs become an even more important source of this vital building block.

It is always best to eat meat and eggs that came from pasture raised animals that were fed a diet similar to what they would eat in the wild. Always stay away from meats that have added preservatives or flavor enhancers, like nitrites or MSG. All different fish species are healthy choices, just be conscious of high mercury levels and choose fish with ecologically friendly harvesting practices. Here are some options: Turkey, chicken, goat, lamb, pork, organ meat (liver, gizzards, heart), game meats (pheasant, duck, deer, bison, goose, quail), beef, eggs (from chicken, duck, emu, etc), fish, shell fish, and fish eggs.

Nuts, Seeds, and Butters: All nuts and seeds are good, as well as the butters made from them. Keep in mind that peanuts are NOT nuts. They are legumes, and thus are NOT part of the Paleo diet. Almond butter makes a great replacement for peanut butter, and there are many mild nut butters that work well in baking.

Fats and Oils: Use fats and oils sparingly. Remember that you can not use grain oils, like corn oil or peanut oil. But there are a lot of great substitutes: lard, tallow, bacon grease, olive oil, coconut oil, walnut oil, avocado oil, hazelnut oil, flaxseed oil (unheated).

Drinks: Filtered or spring water should be your main drink. You can also add herbal tea, coconut water, and freshly juiced fruits and vegetables. Stay away from soda, bottled juice and juice drinks.

Seasoning: Most spices are fine, including sea salt (NOT refined iodized salt).

The following foods/beverages are okay in moderation, but you don't want to overdo them: Coffee, chocolate, caffeinated tea, raw honey, stevia, agave, grade B maple syrup.

FOODS TO AVOID

This is going to be a tough transition for some children, as they are going to have to give up some foods that they love, like cheese, pasta, and bread. But once you start cooking some of the delicious recipes in this book, they will get used to a new, healthier way of eating. They'll start to feel good, and they will stop missing the pizza and sodas!

Cereal Grains: Wheat, rice, barley, corn millet, spelt, kamut, rice, amaranth, sorghum, rye, oats, quinoa, or anything made out of grains (flour, noodles, bread, crackers).

Legumes: All beans are out of the picture, including soybeans (tofu, too) and peanuts. Eliminate black beans, pintos, lentils, peas, lima beans, black-eyed peas, garbanzo beans (hummus), kidney beans, etc.

Sugar and Artificial Sweeteners: white sugar, brown sugar, turbinado sugar, refined maple syrup, high fructose corn syrup, corn syrup, molasses, refined honey, sucralose, aspartame, Splenda, Equal.

Highly Processed Oils and Most Vegetable Oils: Any oil that comes from a seed or legume is not acceptable, like soybean oil, corn oil, safflower oil, and grape seed oil. Also stay away from hydrogenated, partially hydrogenated and refined oils.

Dairy Products: This includes butter, yogurt, cheese and milk from cows, goats, sheep and buffalo. Basically, if it comes from an animal's teat, it is not allowed on the diet. However, that is up for debate in the Paleo community. Do your research. If you choose to eat some dairy, make sure that it is full-fat, raw (unpasteurized), organic and grass-fed, fermented dairy.

FROM ONE PALEO PARENT TO ANOTHER

When my son transitioned to a Paleo diet, I can honestly say that I was surprised at how easy it went. It helps that he is an adventurous eater. But my daughter was very picky, so I picked up a few tricks to make the switch easier for her.

- Play to their strengths. If your child loves apples and almond butter, let them eat it once a day. If they have no problem with vegetables, give them a healthy serving with every meal. If they'll only eat white foods, make it whipped cauliflower and almond chicken fingers. Don't force the weird stuff on them... well, at least not right away.

- Involve them in the kitchen. This step is essential for the long-term health of your children. If they can cook well-balanced Paleo meals that taste great, they will be able to nourish their own bodies for the rest of their lives.

- If your child is very small, they can wash and scrub fruits and veggies. By about the age of three, they could use a crinkle cutter knife that does not cut fingers to help chop carrots, celery, bananas, melon and more. At this age, they can also mix batters, set the table and toss the salads.

- Once they get a bit older, teach them how to hold a knife properly - placing their left hand on top of the knife as they use their right hand to cut (or vice versa for lefties). This way they can cut more difficult things like cooked meats.

- By about the age of eight, they should be able to use the stove to cook a simple scrambled egg and even more elaborate meals. Make sure you are nearby to monitor, though. Have them cook breakfast for the family one day a week. They will be proud of themselves, which makes cooking and eating even more fun.

- Teens should be able to cook entire meals. Make it exciting for them by video recording a "cooking show" that they create themselves.

Let them host a cooking competition with their friends. Have them cater their own party, just for fun! Let them cook a meal for grandma and grandpa. The possibilities are endless here, and you are giving them the gift of a lifetime of healthy eating.

• Let them eat dessert! If your child is used to eating a lot of sweets, they may be feeding a yeast problem, which often shows up as sugar addiction. They'll have to break the cycle, but do it slowly. When you are first starting the Paleo diet, let them have as many of the sweet foods on the approved list as possible. Make the raw brownies and key lime pie. Let them have the avocado chocolate pudding for breakfast with sliced bananas. Pack trail mix with plenty of raisins and dried blueberries in their lunch box. If they don't feel suddenly deprived, they'll be much more open to the idea of changing how they eat and you can slowly taper off the sweets.

• Make it a family affair. Have a family meeting where you talk about the importance of healthy eating. Make the decision to eat like "cavemen" together as a team. You can even turn it into a challenge if your family likes that kind of thing. But any way you approach the switch, do it as an entire family rather than singling out one child to be different. Finally, eat meals together as much as possible.

TOOLS OF THE TRADE

While I'm sure our Paleolithic ancestors did fine without them, there are a few culinary tools and appliances that are indispensable in our modern day Paleo kitchens. While you don't have to have the following items, they will certainly make your life easier.

TOOLS:
- Food processor
- Slow cooker
- Ice cream maker
- Hand mixer
- Parchment paper

FOOD STAPLES:
- Raw honey
- Almonds/nuts
- Grade B maple syrup
- Avocados
- Raw cocoa powder
- Lemon juice
- Coconut oil
- Olive oil
- A wide variety of spices

BREAKFAST MENU

- Apple Cinnamon Noatmeal -
- Bacon Power Plate -
- Blueberry Almond Mini Muffins -
- Farmer's Omelet -
- Fluffy Paleo Pancakes -

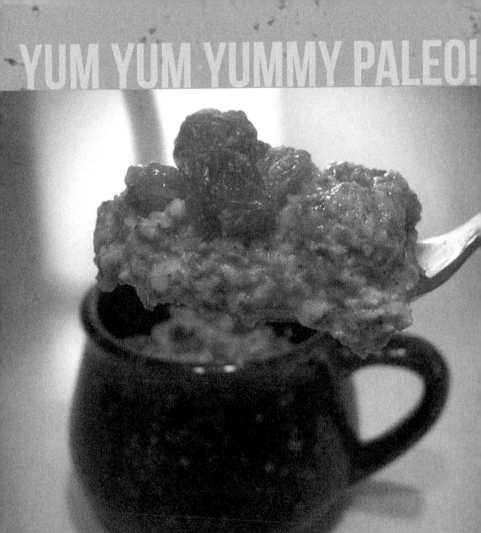

Apple Cinnamon Noatmeal

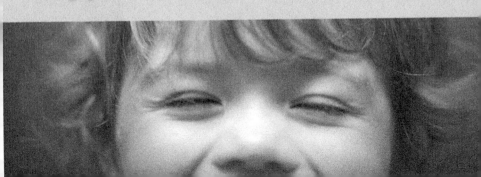

APPLE CINNAMON NOATMEAL

My daughter always loved oatmeal with diced apples and cinnamon on a cold winter morning. It's something we missed when we first started the Paleo diet... until I came up with this delicious substitute. With all the flavors and textures of oatmeal, it warms you and makes you feel all yummy inside.

Apple Cinnamon Noatmeal Recipe

Ingredients:
- ½ cup pecans
- ½ cup almonds
- ½ cup unsweetened almond milk
- 1 apple (any variety)
- 1 teaspoon ground cinnamon
- Grade B maple syrup and raisins (optional)

Directions: Peel, core and roughly chop the apple. Combine pecans, almonds, almond milk, apple and cinnamon in the food processor. Process until completely mixed and grainy. This should have the texture of oatmeal!

Transfer to small pot. Heat for about two minutes over medium heat on the stove- stirring continuously.

Pour into two bowls or mugs. Top with a teaspoon of grade B maple syrup and raisins, if desired. This Noatmeal is already sweet, but the maple syrup and raisins add a nice flavor.

Serving size: ¾ cup   Yields: 2 servings
Prep time: 5 min   Cook Time: 2 min
Total: 7 min

YUM YUM YUMMY PALEO!

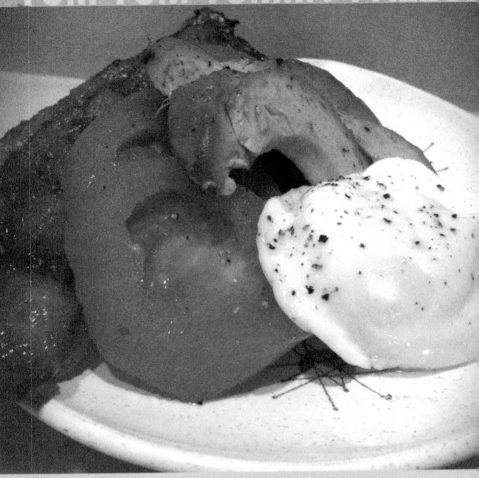

Bacon Power Plate

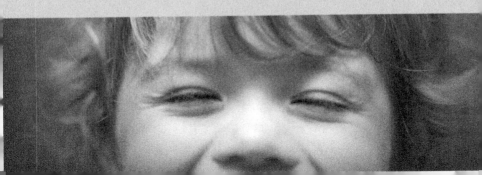

BACON POWER PLATE

The creaminess of the poached egg and avocado perfectly offset the salty crunch of the bacon. The cool, juicy, slightly sweet Roma tomato rounds out this simple breakfast dish. You can serve this simply on the plate, stacked up high, or cut into chunks for smaller children. Any way you slice it, this breakfast is power packed and full of healthy protein.

Bacon Power Plate Recipe

Ingredients:
- 8 slices thick cut bacon
- 4 small Roma tomatoes
- 4 eggs
- 1 avocado
- Freshly ground black pepper

Directions: To make perfect bacon every time, lay out the bacon in strips on a foil-lined rimmed baking sheet. Preheat the oven to 400°F. Bake 10-15 minutes until desired crispness. Time will depend on the thickness of your bacon.

While the bacon is baking, wash and slice the tomatoes into ¼ inch thick slices. To make a good poached egg, you should do them one at a time. Crack your egg into a small bowl or cup. In a small pot, bring a few inches of water to a simmer. Once simmering, with bubbles barely forming around the edges, make a whirlpool in the water with a spoon or spatula. Carefully slide the egg into the center of the whirlpool. It will look messy, but should pull together quickly. You can use a slotted spoon to gently tap stray bits of egg back into place. Let cook for 3 – 4 minutes until whites are firm but yolk is still runny. Remove from water to a plate.

Don't forget to take the bacon out of the oven! Repeat the steps to make all four eggs. Peel and slice the avocado. Arrange all ingredients on four plates and sprinkle with freshly grated pepper. *If the thought of making poached eggs is daunting to you, this recipe easily accommodates fried, scrambled, or soft-boiled eggs.

Serving size: 1 egg, 1 slices of bacon, 1 tomato, ¼ avocado
Yields: 4 servings   Prep time: 10 min
Cook time: 22 min   Total: 32 min

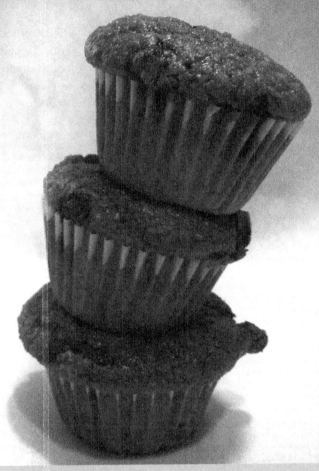

Blueberry Almond Mini Muffins

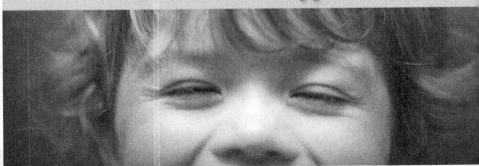

BLUEBERRY ALMOND MINI MUFFINS

These little muffins are great for breakfast. But they're also perfect for bite-sized snacks at the park, for a treat when hosting play dates, or as a side dish in the lunch box. I like to use frozen, thawed blueberries so that I can mix the juice into the batter. But fresh work well, too. Slightly nutty and sweet, everyone will enjoy these berry-packed pastries.

Blueberry Almond Mini Muffin Recipe

Ingredients:
- 1 cup almond meal
- ½ cup ground pecans or pecan meal
- ¾ cup coconut flour
- ½ cup almond milk
- 2 tbsp coconut oil, melted
- 3 eggs
- ½ cup raw honey (or more if you like them very sweet)
- 1 cup blueberries (frozen-thawed or fresh)
- 1 tsp cinnamon
- 1 tsp vanilla
- 1 tsp baking soda (optional)*

Directions: Preheat oven to 350°. In a large bowl, combine the almond meal, pecan meal, coconut flour, cinnamon and baking soda. To the flour mix, add almond milk, coconut oil, eggs, vanilla and honey. Beat batter until smooth and tiny bubbles form on the top of the mixture. With a spoon, stir in blueberries.

Line two one-dozen muffin tins with paper liners. Spoon batter evenly into tins. Bake at 350° 15 – 17 minutes until muffins are fluffy, golden, and a toothpick inserted into center comes out clean. Cool five minutes before removing from pan.

*Baking soda is not necessarily Paleo, but is found in a lot of Paleo baking recipes. It provides a little lift to muffins and cakes, and the amount used is not significant. However, these muffins will turn out fine without it. They will just be denser, more chewy like a pancake. It's your choice depending on how strict you are on your diet.

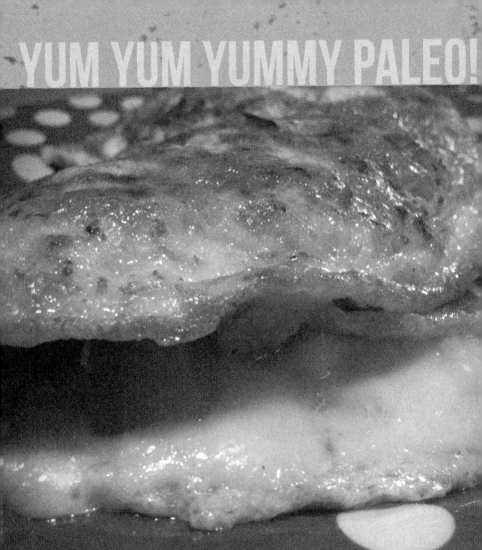

Farmer's Omelet

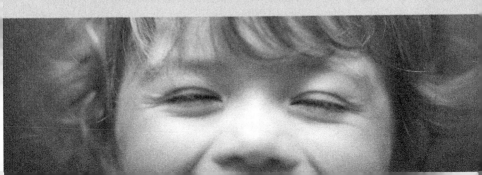

FARMER'S OMELET

This hearty omelet is a great way to start the day. It's protein-packed to fill up hungry bellies, and it's the perfect container for veggies of any kind. You can even use frozen chopped veggie mixes from the grocer's freezer, like tricolored peppers and onions. Or chop a few extras when you're making dinner and stick them in the freezer just for this kind of meal.

Farmer's Omelet Recipe

Ingredients:
- 2 eggs
- 2 slices thick cut bacon
- ½ cup diced frozen (thawed) or fresh vegetables
  If you are chopping fresh vegetables, make sure they are all diced before you begin frying your bacon.
- ¼ tsp garlic powder
- Sea salt and ground black pepper
- Raw cheese (optional)

Directions: In an omelet pan or small nonstick skillet set over medium heat, fry the bacon until chewy but not too done (about 2 minutes on each side).

While the bacon is frying, beat the eggs in a medium sized bowl until frothy. Mix in your vegetables and spices. I used a mixture of frozen (thawed) broccoli, diced onion, and tomato. But use whichever vegetables your kids like best! Remove the bacon to a cutting board, leaving the grease in the pan. Pour the egg mixture into the grease. While the omelet begins to cook, coarsely chop the bacon and sprinkle it over the top of the egg mixture.

When the edges of the omelet start to puff, gently slip a spatula under one edge and lift it. With your other hand, tilt the pan so the runny egg from the top and center of the omelet drains to the outer edge. This will cook your omelet evenly. Repeat this step until the omelet is set in the center. It should cook about five minutes, with three to four lift-and-drains. If you are using raw cheese, sprinkle it across the top once the omelet is set. Fold one side of the omelet over with a spatula. Slide it onto a plate and enjoy a hearty, healthy breakfast.

Serving size: 1 omelet   Yields: 1 serving
Prep time: 5 min   Cook time: 7 – 10 min   Total time: 12 – 15 min

YUM YUM YUMMY PALEO!

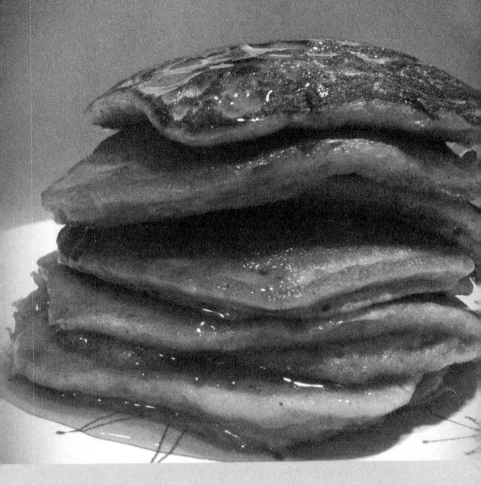

Fluffy Paleo Pancakes

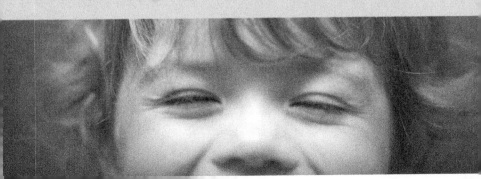

FLUFFY PALEO PANCAKES

When I first made these pancakes, I have to admit that I was skeptical. How can you combine green bananas with egg and make that taste good? Then I took a bite. So did my son. He put down his fork and said what I was thinking... "These are awesome!" You can easily add blueberries, sliced ripe banana and cocoa powder, or even thinly sliced apple and raisins. The batter is simple, so it takes on other flavors nicely.

Fluffy Paleo Pancakes Recipe

Ingredients:
- 2 under-ripe bananas (mostly green with a little yellow)
- 2 eggs
- 1 ½ tbsp coconut oil plus more for frying
- 1 tsp vanilla
- 1 tsp cinnamon (or to taste)
- Grade B Maple Syrup or other toppings

Directions: Combine all ingredients in a blender. Blend on high until smooth and bubbly. Heat oil for frying (about one tablespoon) in a non-stick skillet set over medium to high heat or an electric griddle.

When the oil is sizzling, pour batter in small pools (about two tablespoons each) on the pan. Cook until the center of the pancake bubbles and the edges pull away from the pan. Flip, and cook until the pancake is cooked through the middle and golden on both sides. Remove to a plate and top with grade B maple syrup.

Serving size: 3 pancakes   Yields: 2 servings
Prep time: 5 min   Cook time: 5 min
Total time: 10 minutes

LUNCH MENU

- Chicken Fingers -
- Sweet Potato Fries -
- Grandma's Chicken Soup -
- Dinosaur Eggs -
- Almond Cookie Tart -
- Beef And Asparagus Rolls -
- Roasted Eggplant Dip With Veggies -

YUM YUM YUMMY PALEO!

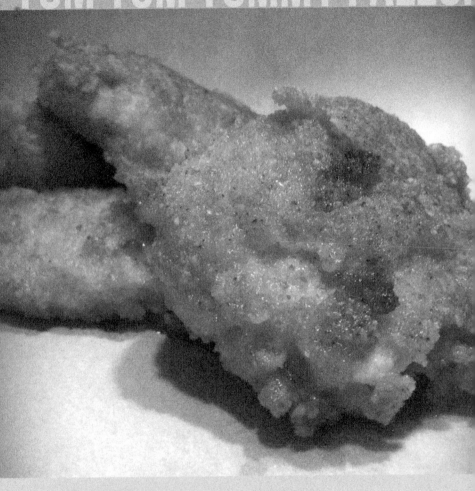

Chicken Fingers

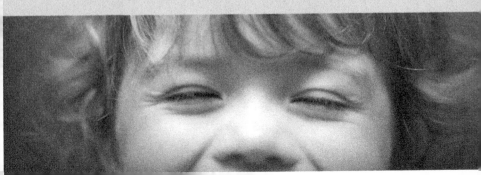

CHICKEN FINGERS

I'll be the first to admit that a quick meal of chicken nuggets and fries is something I take comfort in on those long days when cooking doesn't sound as fun as it usually is for our family! (Or when I'm craving junk food.) Here's the good news: With a little prep work, you can have the convenience of those meals when you need them! This chicken recipe can be made ahead in large batches and frozen. Just pull it out and bake however many you need!

Chicken Fingers Recipe

Ingredients:
- 2 large chicken breasts (boneless, skinless)
- 1 cup blanched almond meal
- 2 eggs
- 1 tsp paprika
- 1 tsp garlic powder
- ¼ cup olive oil
- Salt to taste

Directions: On a cutting board, slice your chicken breasts into thin strips. Set aside. In a medium sized bowl, beat the two eggs until the yolk and whites are whipped together. In another bowl, mix the almond meal with the spices. Start the olive oil over medium heat in a large heavy skillet.

Dunk the chicken strips into the egg mixture, and then into the almond meal mixture to coat. Once coated, place directly into the hot oil. Fry until golden brown and center is cooked through, and then flip to fry the other side. (3-5 minutes each side).

You may have to do this in several batches. You can put each batch in a 350° oven, on an foil-lined pan, while you finish cooking all the chicken. Serve immediately with raw honey mustard dip, or place into glass containers with lids and stick right in the freezer. When you're ready to heat-and-eat, simply place the frozen nuggets on a foil-lined pan. Bake at 325° for 22 – 27 minutes until heated through.

Serving size: 5 strips   Yields: 4 servings
Prep time: 10 min   Cook time: 20 min   Total time: 30 min

YUM YUM YUMMY PALEO!

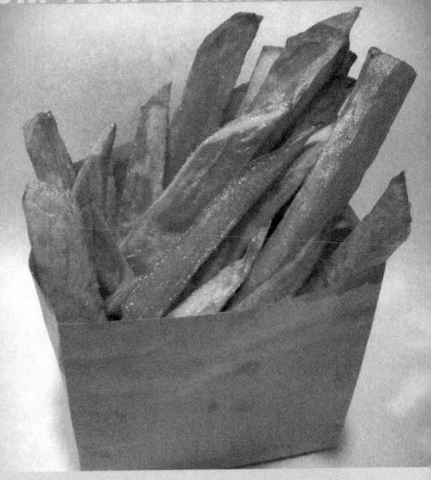

Sweet Potato Fries

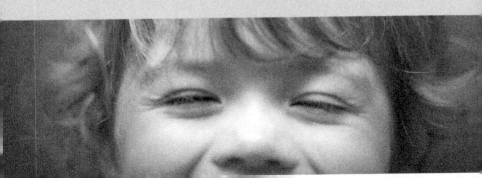

SWEET POTATO FRIES

Okay, I'll let you in on a dirty little secret... My kids and I are french fry junkies. We love them with chicken, or burgers, or by themselves dunked in catsup or honey mustard. On the Paleo diet, we try to limit our intake of white potatoes. Even though they are technically allowed, they are kind of empty calories. But we can still get our fry fix by substituting nutrient-rich sweet potatoes for the starchy white tubers.

Sweet Potato Fries Recipe

Ingredients:
- 1 large sweet potato
- 1 quart olive oil

Directions: In a medium heavy pot, or a deep fryer, heat the oil until it's very hot, about ten minutes. While it's heating, peel the sweet potato and remove bad spots. Slice into desired shapes with a very sharp knife.

Carefully drop the fries into the hot oil. Be careful, the oil may splatter or pop. Fry until the fries are golden and crisp. The time can vary based on the size of cut, the heat of the oil, and the size of the pan. Just watch them carefully. It should take 5 to 7 minutes.

With a slatted spoon, remove fries to a plate covered with paper towel. Shake on sea salt to taste. Let cool for a few minutes before serving.

TO MAKE SWEET POTATO CHIPS: Use the same recipe, but instead of cutting into fry shapes, use a mandolin or very sharp knife to slice the potatoes paper thin. Fry in the oil for about 2 – 4 minutes.

These fries can be frozen and heated in the oven later. Simply spread them out on a parchment lined baking pan and freeze until they're frozen through. Then empty them into a zip-top bag. When ready to use, bake them in a 350° oven for about 15 minutes or until heated through and crisp.

*You can save the oil in a mason jar to use again for your next batch of fries!

Serving size: ½ potato   Yields: 2 servings
Prep time: 5 min   Cook time: 7 min   Total time: 12 min

YUM YUM YUMMY PALEO!

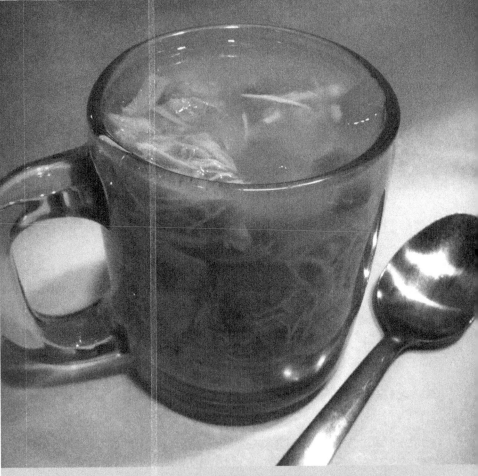

Grandma's Chicken Soup

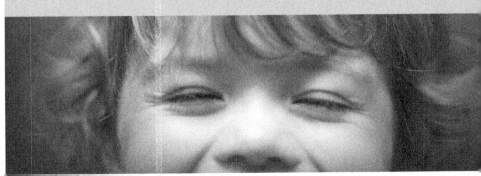

GRANDMA'S CHICKEN SOUP

My grandma always made the best chicken soup. She'd boil the chicken all day, pull it out and strip it of its meat, then return it to the pot with celery, carrots and fresh parsley. Just before eating it, she'd add eggs noodles. This recipe has all the same mouth-watering qualities of grandma's best comfort food, but it skips the noodles- and the "all day" part! Honestly, neither one is missed.

Grandma's Chicken Soup Recipe

Ingredients:
- 1 pound chicken or more. This can be from a roasted chicken, chicken breast and thighs, or a boiled chicken just for the soup.
- 6 cups chicken stock
- 1 celery stalk
- 1 carrot
- 1 tbsp chopped fresh parsley
- Salt and pepper to taste

Directions: Strip the chicken from bones and pull apart into shreds. Wash and chop the celery and carrot. Place the vegetables in a large pot with the chicken stock. Boil for 5 – 7 minutes until the celery and carrots are tender. Reduce heat to simmer. Add chicken, salt, pepper and parsley. Simmer until soup is heated through, about 3 minutes.

This soup is perfect as is, but if you're dead set on noodles, you can rinse and add a cup of kelp noodles and simmer for another two minutes until noodles are soft. Keep in mind: While the kelp noodles are delicious and healthy, they are a lot chewier than regular noodles and may not please picky eaters.

Serving size: 1 cup   Yields: 8 servings
Prep time: 10 min   Cook time: 10 min
Total time: 17 min

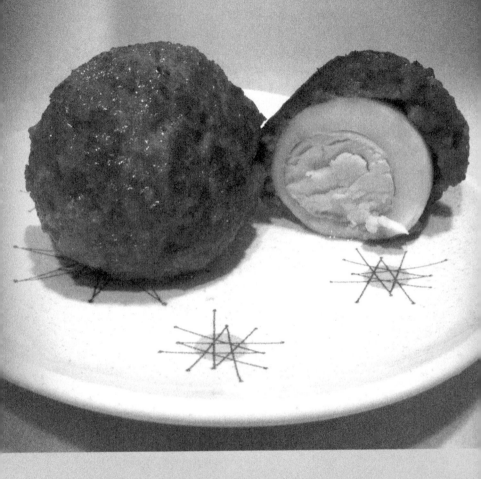

YUM YUM YUMMY PALEO!

Dinosaur Eggs

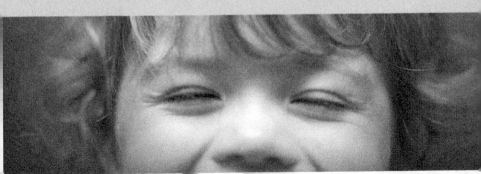

DINOSAUR EGGS

What better for a Caveman diet than these protein-packed dinosaur eggs? They're really just scotch eggs, the delicious sausage-wrapped treats my kids look forward to munching on every time we go to a Renaissance Festival. Then I discovered how easy they are to make! Served with catsup or honey-mustard, these savory finger foods quickly became a lunch-box staple.

Dinosaur Egg Recipe

Ingredients:
- 1 ½ pounds ground sausage
- 6 eggs
- Olive oil or bacon grease for frying

Directions: First, boil the eggs. Place eggs in a two quart pot. Cover them with water and bring to a boil. Immediately remove from heat, cover and let sit twenty minutes. Plunge in cold water. Peel the eggs, discarding shell. Preheat oven to 400°F.

Divide the sausage into six equal portions. Flatten sausage into rounds. Place an egg in the middle of a sausage round and carefully wrap the sausage around the egg, making sure there are no holes. The sausage should be very thick around the egg, because it will shrink when it cooks and you don't want to end up with a "cracked" coating.

Pour about a centimeter of oil or grease into a large skillet set over medium heat. When it starts to sizzle and pop, gently add in the sausage-wrapped eggs. Fry until the face down side is golden brown, and then rotate with a slotted spoon until all sides are done. Remove to a rimmed cookie sheet.

Place in oven for 8 – 10 minutes until the sausage is cooked through. Serve with catsup or honey-mustard dip.

*I always make a double batch of these dinosaur eggs so I have them in the refrigerator for lunches or outings. They are just as good cold!

Serving size: 1 egg   Yields: 6 servings
Prep Time (including boiling) 30 min   Cook Time: 20 min   Total: 50 min

YUM YUM YUMMY PALEO!

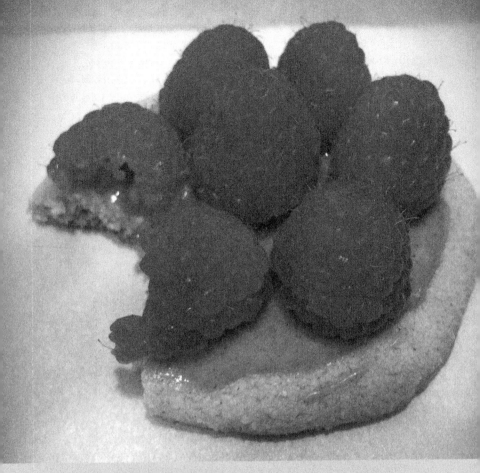

Almond Cookie Tart

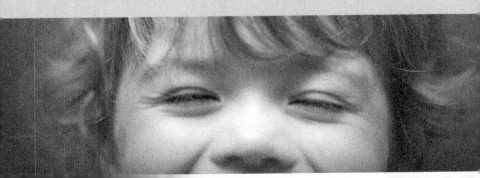

ALMOND COOKIE TART

My children used to love peanut butter and jelly sandwiches. When we started the Paleo diet, I didn't want them to miss out on the foods they loved, so I came up with this tart that mimics the flavors of a PBJ! If you keep these almond cookies on hand (see Almond Cookie recipe), which I do, this lunch is a snap!

Almond Cookie Tart Recipe

Ingredients:
- 1 almond cookie (see recipe)
- 1 tsp almond butter (or nut butter of choice)
- 7 raspberries

Directions: Spread the nut butter evenly over the cookie. Rinse and pat dry the raspberries. Set them on top of the nut butter. Enjoy!

Serving size: 1 tart   Yields: 1 serving
Prep time: 3 minutes   Cook time: 0
Total: 3 minutes

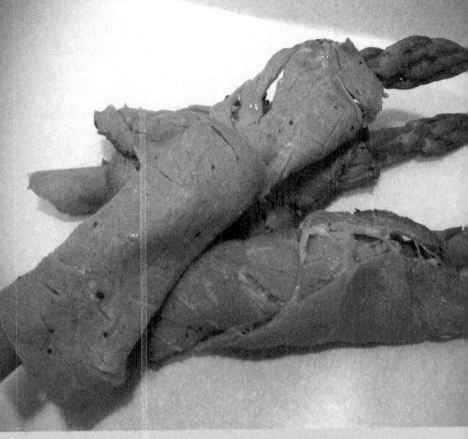

Beef And Asparagus Rolls

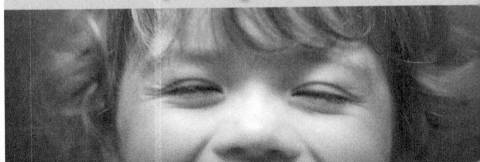

BEEF AND ASPARAGUS ROLLS

The sweet and tangy honey mustard, combined with the rich flavors of roast beef and the light snap of parboiled asparagus make this lunch a hit with everyone in our house! You can even try substituting different fruits, vegetables, and sauces to shake things up a bit. Set the meats, veggies, and dips out and let your kids make their own creations! How about sliced chicken wrapped around a thin carrot stick with Paleo catsup? I like roasted turkey with honey mustard around a sliced cucumber. The possibilities are endless.

Beef and Asparagus Roll Recipe

Ingredients:
- 3 asparagus spears
- 3 thick slices roast beef
- 1 tsp honey mustard

Directions: In a small pan, heat about two cups of water to boiling. As you wait, rinse the asparagus and trim off the fibrous ends. Drop the trimmed asparagus into the boiling water for about thirty seconds. Remove with tongs and rinse immediately with cold water to stop the cooking. You want these parboiled, crisp in the middle and slightly cooked on the outside.

Open the three slices of beef on a plate. Divide the honey mustard sauce evenly between the slices. Place one asparagus spear at the end of each slice of beef, and roll tightly. *Alternately, you can serve the honey mustard sauce on the side for dipping.

Serving size: 3 rolls   Yields: 1 serving
Prep time: 7 min   Cook time: 30 sec
Total: 7 ½ min

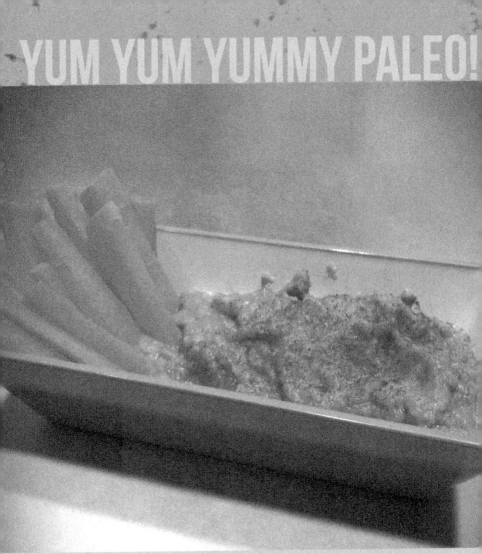

Roasted Eggplant Dip With Veggies

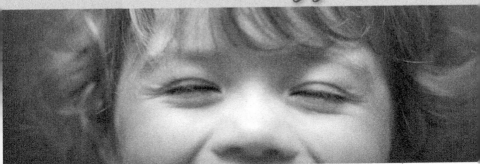

ROASTED EGGPLANT DIP WITH VEGGIES

This dip is traditionally called baba ghanouj, a middle eastern dish similar in flavor and texture to its more popular cousin- hummus! I have it here on the lunch menu because we will often grab it out of the fridge with a tub of cut veggies or some sweet potato chips for a quick midday meal. But this dip is equally good spread on grilled meats.

Roasted Eggplant Dip with Veggies Recipe

Ingredients:
- 1 medium eggplant
- 1 – 2 cloves garlic, peeled
- 1 tbsp lemon juice
- 3 tsp extra virgin olive oil
- ¼ tsp cumin
- Smoked paprika, for serving (optional)
- Salt and pepper to taste

Directions: Preheat oven to 425°F. Prick eggplant a dozen or so times with a fork. Set it on a rimmed baking dish. Bake for 35 – 40 minutes until skin is wilted and flesh is soft. Remove from dish with tongs and plunge into a large bowl of cold water.

When eggplant is cool enough to handle, cut off the stem. Peel off the skin and discard. Cut the flesh into chunks.

Place all the ingredients into a food processor. Process on high until mixture is uniform, but still slightly lumpy. Remove to a bowl. Sprinkle with paprika (if desired) and serve warm or cold with cut veggies or sweet potato chips.

DINNER MENU

- *Meatloaf Muffins* -
- *Whipped Cauliflower* -
- *Taco Wraps* -
- *Beef And Baby Bella Sticks* -
- *Chopped Chicken Stir Fry* -
- *Slow Cooker Sweet Potato Casserole* -

YUM YUM YUMMY PALEO!

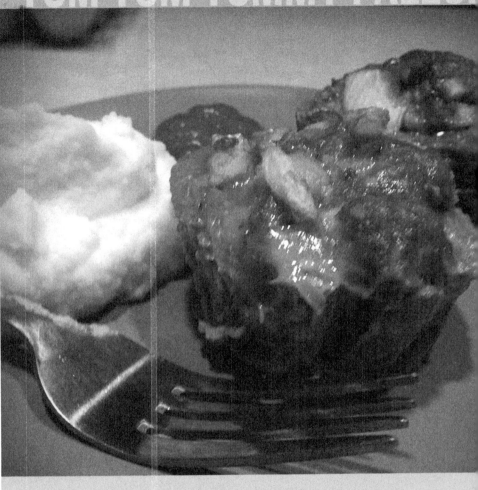

Meatloaf Muffins

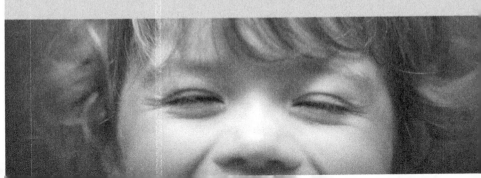

MEATLOAF MUFFINS

This kid-friendly Paleo version of meatloaf is delicious, healthy, and fun! You can pair it with whipped cauliflower for a traditional "meatloaf and mashed potatoes" dinner, or serve it with Paleo catsup and sweet potato fries for a fun finger food meal. These protein packed savory "muffins" are also good cold, as a simple addition to the lunch box or picnic basket.

Meatloaf Muffin Recipe

Ingredients:
- 1 lb lean ground beef or bison
- 1 small yellow onion
- 2 eggs
- ½ cup almond meal
- ½ tsp garlic powder
- ½ tsp dried basil
- Sea salt and pepper to taste

Directions: Preheat oven to 350°F. Peel and finely dice the yellow onion. Place all ingredients into a large bowl. Squish and turn with your hands until the mixture has an even consistency. Kids love to do this job, but make sure they wash their hands with soap and water before they dig in, and as soon as they are done!

Scoop by the 1/3 cup into a regular sized muffin pan until all the mixture has been used. Place pan into the preheated oven. Bake 25 – 30 minutes until the meatloaf muffins are firm to the touch and a meat thermometer inserted into the center reads at least 160°. Remove to a trivet and let rest five minutes. Remove with a serving fork.

Serving size: 2 Meatloaf Muffins   Yields: 4 – 5 servings
Prep time: 5 min   Cook time: 25 – 30 min
Total time: 30 – 35 min

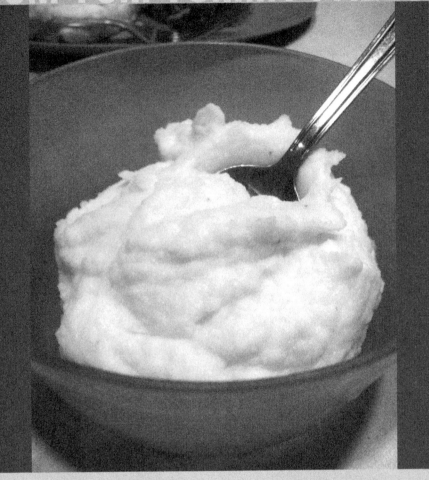

Whipped Cauliflower

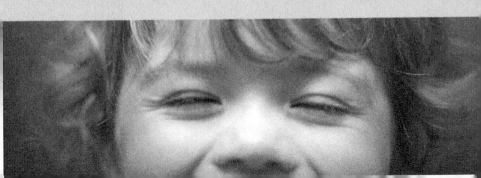

WHIPPED CAULIFLOWER

Whipped cauliflower is a quick, simple replacement for traditional mashed potatoes. Serve them with meatloaf muffins, roasted chicken, grilled steaks, or skillet pork chops. Kids love the mild flavor and smooth texture.

Whipped Cauliflower Recipe

Ingredients:
- 1 head organic cauliflower
- 2 – 4 cloves roasted garlic (optional)
- 3 tbsp olive oil
- Sea salt and pepper to taste

Directions: Set a large pot of water (with a steamer basket) over the stove set to high heat. While you wait for the water to boil, prepare cauliflower. Remove stem and leaves. Wash and shake dry. Roughly chop the cauliflower into large pieces. Place chopped cauliflower into the steamer basket. Set steamer basket over boiling water and cover with lid. Allow to steam until very soft, about 15 minutes. When cauliflower is completely done, place it into a food processor with garlic, olive oil, salt and pepper. Process until smooth and fluffy, 2 – 4 minutes.

Serving size: ½ cup   Yields: 4 – 5 servings
Prep time: 7 min   Cook time: 15 min
Total time: 22 min

YUM YUM YUMMY PALEO!

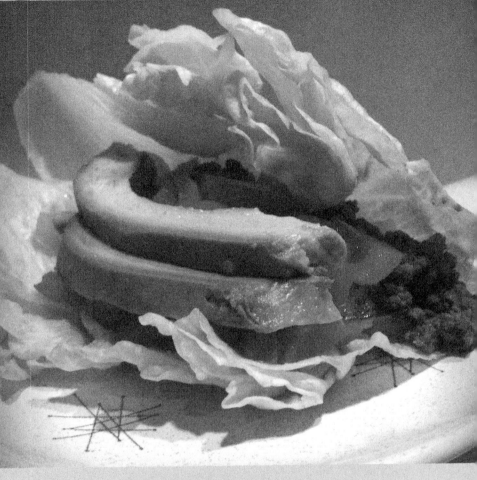

Taco Wraps

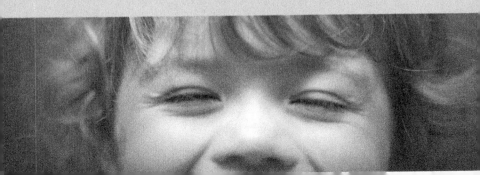

TACO WRAPS

Taco night is a family tradition stemming from my own childhood. Every Friday night my dad would season and cook the meat while my brother and I chopped vegetables and set the table. My own kids love this tradition. We put all the ingredients on a large serving platter on a lazy susan in the middle of the table, and we assemble our own tacos as we chat and laugh and eat!

Taco Wrap Recipe

Ingredients:
- 1 lb ground beef
- 1 head iceberg lettuce
- 1 tomato
- 2 peppers (yellow, green, red- choose two)
- 1 small onion
- 1 tsp cumin
- 1 tsp garlic powder
- 1 tsp chili powder (or smoked paprika)
- 1 tbsp olive oil
- Salt and pepper to taste
- 1 avocado, sliced (for topping)
- Cilantro (garnish)

Directions: Dice the vegetables (except avocado). In a large pan over medium heat, brown ground beef with spices, about 8 minutes. In another pan, heat olive oil over medium-high heat. Toss in vegetables and saute until just cooked, about five minutes. Slice avocado and dice tomato.

Rinse head of lettuce, peeling away any flimsy outside layers. Cut horizontally down the center. Use the "top" slices as cups for your taco wraps. Pile the lettuce cups with meat and vegetables. Top with avocado slices and fresh cilantro. Fold over and enjoy!

Serving Size: 2 taco wraps   Yields: 5 servings
Prep Time: 10 min   Cook Time: 13 – 15 minutes
Total: 25 min

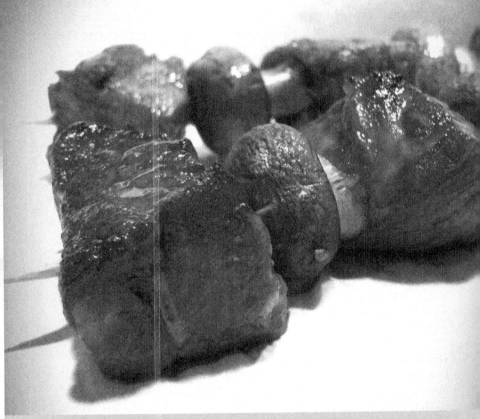

Beef And Baby Bella Sticks

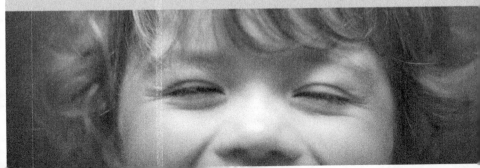

BEEF AND BABY BELLA STICKS

Nothing is better for kids than a meal you can eat with your fingers! This is a simple meat and mushroom kebab that is delicious and easy to prepare. All the marinade ingredients go right into a large zip-top bag, so there's not a lot of fuss in the kitchen. In the summer, I make these on the grill. But in the winter or on rainy days, I use this broiler method.

Beef and Baby Bella Sticks Recipe

Ingredients:

- 2 lbs lean beef steak cut into 1" cubes (you can substitute bison or lamb)
- 12 oz baby portobella mushrooms
- ¼ cup Coconut Aminos*
- ¼ cup raw honey
- 1 large clove garlic, crushed

Directions: Line a jelly roll pan with aluminum foil. Gently wash mushrooms and set aside. In a large zip-top plastic bag, combine coconut aminos, honey and garlic. Zip the top of the bag tight and shake until the marinade is mixed well.

Open the bag and add the meat and mushrooms. Seal the bag and shake again until everything is coated. At this point, you can go ahead and cook the kebabs, or let the meat and mushrooms marinade up to twenty-four hours.

Preheat the broiler to high. Slide mushrooms and steak onto wood or metal skewers, alternating between meat and mushrooms. Lay the full skewers down on the aluminum lined pan with all the "handle's" on one side. Slide the pan under the broiler with "handles" facing out.

Broil approximately eight minutes. With an oven mitt (because the skewers will be hot), turn them over using the "handles." Broil another eight minutes until the mushrooms are wilted and juicy and the meat is done to your liking.

Remove from the oven and let cool for a few minutes before plating. Serve with cut raw vegetables, a field green salad, or with sweet potato fries and Paleo catsup for a heartier meal.

*Coconut Aminos are a grain and soy free substitute for tamari or soy sauce. You can find it at most health food stores.

Serving size: 2 sticks   Yields: 4 servings
Prep time: 10 min   Cook time: 16 – 20 min   Total time: 30 min

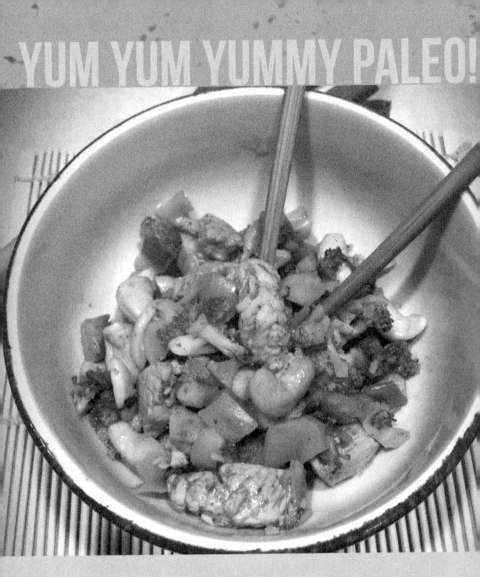

YUM YUM YUMMY PALEO!

Chopped Chicken Stirfry

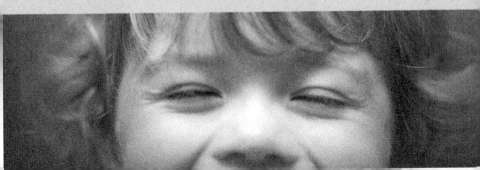

CHOPPED CHICKEN STIR FRY

Kids love chopsticks! This Asian-inspired stir fry is a perfect meal for mastering the use of these difficult dining tools. Sometimes my kids will abandoned the tricky sticks and finish off their meal with a fork. But it's still fun to try, especially when the meal is this good. Chinese five-spice powder provides a nice sweet-n-tangy flavor while the cashews give it a nutty crunch. Since it's all chopped up in tiny pieces, this stir fry also makes a perfect lettuce wrap!

Chopped Chicken Stir Fry Recipe

Ingredients:
- 2 boneless, skinless chicken breasts
- 2 cups chopped broccoli
- 1 cup cashews
- 2 tbsp Coconut Aminos
- 2 tbsp lemon juice
- 1 tsp Chinese five spice powder
- 2 cloves garlic, crushed
- 2 tbsp olive or coconut oil
- 5 green onions

Directions: Finely chop the raw chicken and set aside. In a medium sized bowl, whisk together the Coconut Aminos, lemon juice, five spice powder and garlic. Soak chicken in the sauce while you chop the broccoli and green onion. In a large skillet or wok, heat the oil over high heat. Add in the chicken with all of the marinade. Cook, stirring constantly, for about 5 minutes until the chicken is nearly cooked through. Add in the broccoli and cook another 3 – 5 minutes until broccoli is tender. Add in cashews and green onion and continue cooking for about 12 minutes until all the vegetables are tender and the dish is heated through.

Remove to bowls or lettuce cups and serve immediately.

Serving size: 1 cup   Yields: 4 servings
Prep time: 10 min Cook time: 12 min
Total: 22 min

YUM YUM YUMMY PALEO!

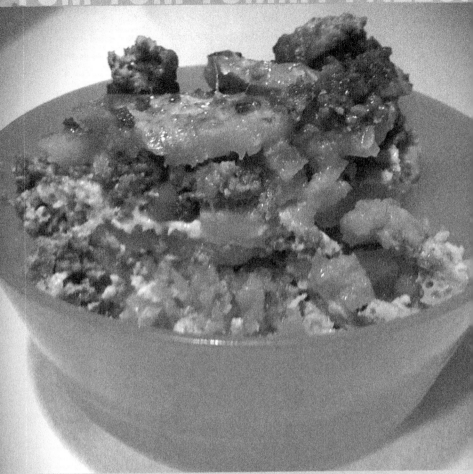

Slow Cooker Sweet Potato Casserole

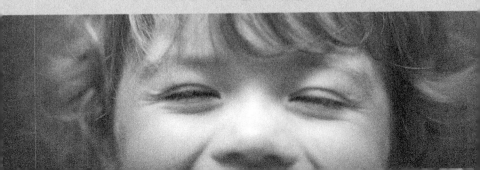

SLOW COOKER SWEET POTATO CASSEROLE

When we are going to have a really busy day, I know that throwing a meal in the slow cooker in the morning can help relieve stress at dinner time, when everyone is tired. This layered casserole perfectly combines sweet and savory in every single bite. It's full of the antioxidant power of sweet potatoes, and the protein that will help your kids build their brains and feel full.

Slow Cooker Sweet Potato Casserole Recipe

Ingredients:
- 2 large sweet potatoes
- 1 lb lean ground beef
- 1 large yellow onion
- 8 eggs
- 1 lb bacon, chopped
- Salt, pepper, and garlic powder to taste

Directions: In a heavy pan, cook the chopped bacon until cooked through but not crispy. Set aside.

Peel and coarsely chop the onion. Peel and slice the potato thin, either with a sharp knife or mandolin. Set aside. In a large pan, cook the onion and ground beef together over medium heat until the meat is browned and the onion is tender, about 5 – 8 minutes.

Crack the eggs into a mixing bowl. Beat with a whisk until mixed through. Spread 1/3 of the bacon, with some of the grease, in the bottom of a two-quart slow cooker. Top the bacon layer with a layer of sweet potatoes, followed by a layer of ground beef and onion mixture. Salt, pepper, and garlic powder the layers as desired. Repeat the process until all of the ingredients are used, making sure to top with the beef- it should take about three layers.

Finally, pour the egg mixture over the top of the casserole. It will sink down in between the layers. Place the lid on the crock pot, and slow cook on low heat for eight hours, or high heat 5 – 6 hours.

Serving size: 1 ½ cups   Yields: 5 – 7 servings
Prep time: (includes cooking bacon and beef) 25 min
Cook time: 5 – 8 hours   Total: 5 hours, 25 min – 8 hours, 25 min

DESSERT MENU

- Almond Sugar Cookies -
- Raw Brownies -
- Chocolate Pudding -
- Fruit Juice Jiggly Dessert -
- Honeyed Honeydew Sorbet -
- Un-Oatmeal Cookies -

YUM YUM YUMMY PALEO!

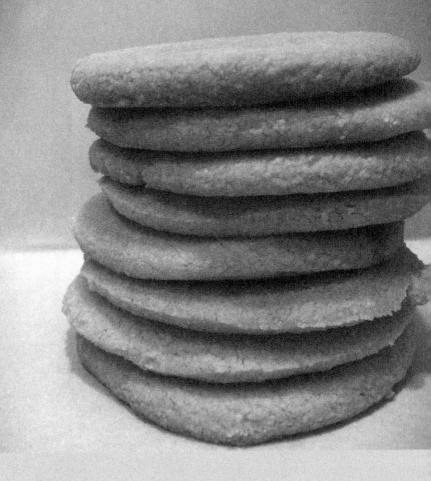

Almond Sugar Cookies

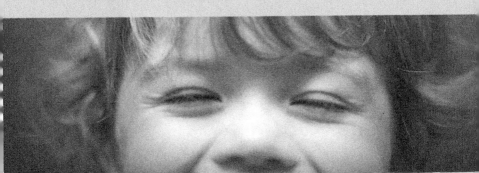

ALMOND SUGAR COOKIES

These are quite simply the best cookies on the planet, Paleo or otherwise. Simple to make and perfectly sweet, these cookies are a versatile, filling and healthy alternative to a bakery treat. We will eat them plain as a snack, as a yummy ending to our meal, or dress them up with nut butters and fruits for lunch. When it's close to the holidays, we'll cut them into snow flake shapes and sprinkle them with a little xylitol for parties or potlucks. Shhhhh... no-one ever guesses these cookies are good for them!

Almond Sugar Cookie Recipe

Ingredients:
- 2 cups blanched almond meal
- 3 tbsp coconut oil
- 3 tbsp raw honey
- ¼ tsp baking soda*
- Dash cinnamon

Directions: Preheat oven to 325°F. In a mixing bowl with an electric beater, or a food processor, combine all ingredients. Mix or process until a thick dough forms, about 3 – 5 minutes. Press dough into a soft ball and set on a sheet of parchment paper.

Place another sheet of parchment paper on top of dough ball. Roll the dough with a rolling pin to desired thickness, about ¼ inch. Cut with a round (or shaped) cookie cutter and place cut cookies on a parchment lined cookie sheet.

When you've cut as many shapes as possible, press remaining scraps of dough back into a ball and re-roll. Repeat this until all the dough has been used. Generally, I use the small-sized mason jar canning ring because it cuts the perfect size for my needs.

Bake about 7 – 9 minutes until the cookies are golden brown. Let cook on the cookie sheet until cooled and set, about five minutes.

*Some Paleo dieters do not use baking soda. You can omit the soda here, but your cookies will be crisp rather than soft and chewy.

Serving size: 1 cookie   Yields: 12 servings
Prep time: 15 min Bake time: 7 – 9 min   Total: 24 min

YUM YUM YUMMY PALEO!

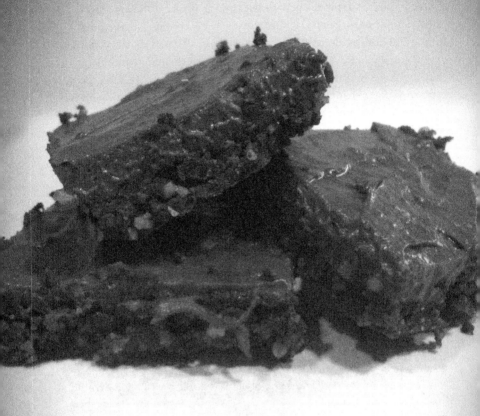

Raw Brownies

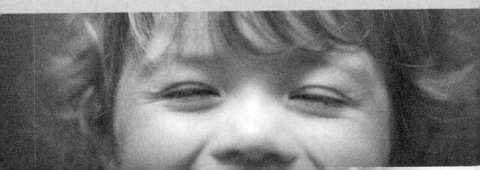

RAW BROWNIES

Could a brownie possibly be healthy? Packed with nuts, dates, and even avocado, these brownies are perfect for a potluck dish, dessert at home, or an energy-filled snack on your way to the park. So chewy and chocolatey, your kids won't even realize these are good for them.

Raw Brownie Recipe

Ingredients:
- 1 cup walnuts (you can substitute pecans, but NOT almonds)
- 1 cup pitted Medjool dates
- 1/3 cup raw cocoa powder

Icing:
- 2 tbsp raw honey
- 2 tbsp raw cocoa powder
- 1 ripe avocado
- 2 tsp vanilla
- Dash of salt and cinnamon (optional)

To make the brownie: Process dates in a food processor until they are finely ground. Add walnuts and cocoa powder. Process again until the nuts are chopped to your taste and the mixture has reached the consistency of potting soil.

Line an 8" x 8" pan with parchment paper. Pour mixture into pan. Press it down into the paper and into the edges of the pan. The more you press, the better your brownie will hold together.

To make the icing: Rinse out your food processor. Slice the avocado around the middle and remove the pit. Scoop out flesh into the food processor. Add the remaining icing ingredients and process until smooth.

Scoop the icing into the brownie. Spread evenly. Cover the pan and place in the freezer for at least an hour. Remove from freezer and cut into squares. Serve immediately or keep frozen, covered, up to two weeks.

Serving size: 1 square   Yields: 12 servings
Prep time: 10 min   Freeze time: 1 hour   Total time: 1 hour, 10 minutes

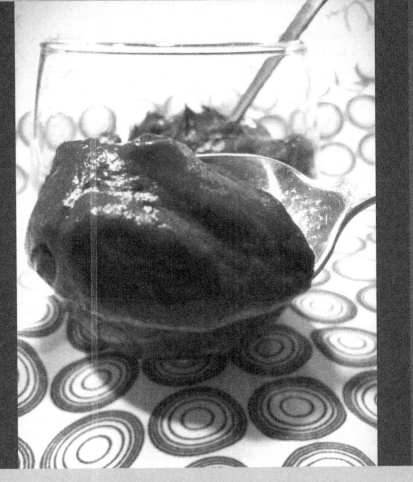

Chocolate Pudding

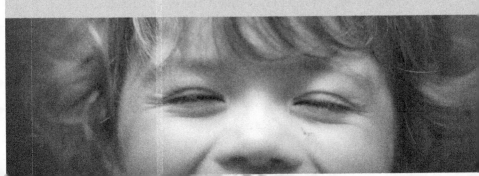

CHOCOLATE PUDDING

Smooth and creamy, this pudding instantly became one of my children's favorite snacks. You can make the recipe in one large bowl, or separate it into small glass containers with lids for pudding packs that drop quickly into lunch boxes.

Chocolate Pudding Recipe

Ingredients:
- Two ripe avocados
- ½ cup cocoa powder
- ½ cup raw honey
- 2 tbsp almond or coconut milk
- ½ teaspoon vanilla

Directions: Slice the avocado in half around the pit. Remove pit and discard. Scrape avocado meat out of the rind and place into a food processor. Add in the remaining ingredients and process until smooth.

Pour into serving bowl, small cups, or small containers with lids for a quick lunch box snack later. Refrigerate if not using immediately.

Serving size: ½ cup   Yields: 4 servings
Prep time: 5 min   Cook time: 0 minutes
Total time: 5 min

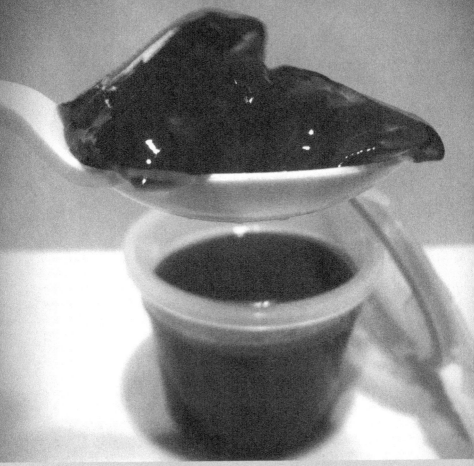

Fruit Juice
Jiggly Dessert

FRUIT JUICE JIGGLY DESSERT

Much like its artificially colored, artificially flavored kid-marketed counterpart, Jello, this jiggly jello dessert is a kid crowd pleaser. But because it doesn't contain any of that bad stuff, moms and dads are happy to let their smiling children have a second helping. You can make it in a jello mold, a large glass bowl, or in individual snack-sized cups. Just remember, if you're packing it in lunches, it has to be kept very cold with ice packs or it will melt into juice (unlike the prepackaged ones you see at the store).

Fruit Juice Jiggly Dessert Recipe

Ingredients:
- 2 cups freshly squeezed juice, any kind (except pineapple)
- 1 7-gram packet plain gelatin

Directions: In a five-cup or larger glass bowl, sprinkle the gelatin on top of ½ cup juice. Heat the remaining juice (1 ½ cups) to boiling in a pot on the stove. Remove from heat. Pour into the bowl with the juice/gelatin mixture. Whisk until all the gelatin has dissolved. Cover and refrigerate at least two hours until set. Serve immediately when removed from the refrigerator plain or topped with berries. If left out, this gelatin dessert will melt.

Serving size: ½ cup   Yields: 4 servings
Prep time: 5 min   Refrigeration time: 2 hours   Total: 2 hours, 5 min

*While strict Paleo diets require that all juices be freshly squeezed from your home juicer, I will often substitute organic unfiltered bottled juices in a pinch.

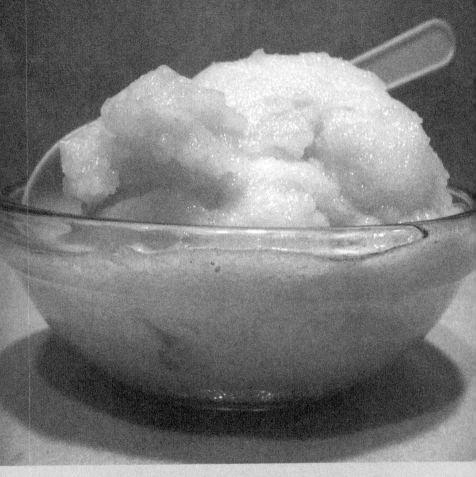

Honeyed Honeydew Sorbet

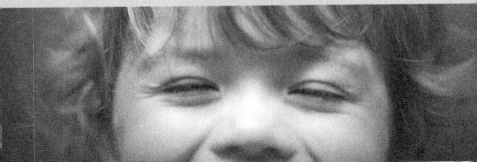

HONEYED HONEYDEW SORBET

One of the best tools in my home kitchen is an ice cream maker. I purchased mine at a big box store for only $29.99. I use it to make slushies and ice cream, sorbet and to make creamy smoothies from freshly blended fruits. This sorbet is light and sweet with just a hint of mint. It's especially good as a dessert after the chicken stir fry.

Honeyed Honeydew Sorbet Recipe

Ingredients:
- 3 cups cubed ripe honeydew melon
- 1 tbsp raw honey
- ¼ tsp peppermint extract (or ½ tsp crushed fresh mint)

Directions: Puree all ingredients in food processor until very smooth. Pour into frozen ice cream maker bucket. Freeze according to your ice cream maker's directions- about 25 minutes. Scoop into cups and serve immediately.

Serving size: ½ cup   Yields: 4 servings
Prep time: 5 min   Freeze time: 25 min
Total: 30 min

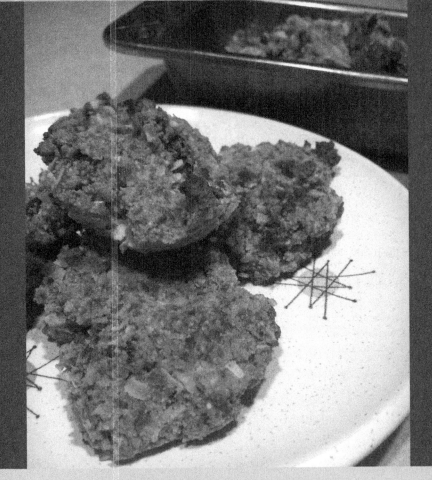

Un-Oatmeal Cookies

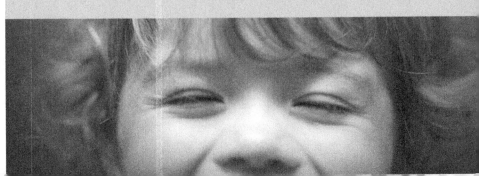

UN-OATMEAL COOKIES

My daughter has never been a big oatmeal cookie fan. But when I made these super-healthy un-oatmeal cookies packed with coconut, pecans and cinnamon, she ate five in a row straight off the cooling rack. The best part is that I didn't care, because I can honestly say this is a dessert that can be eaten before dinner... or for dinner! (Or even for breakfast.)

Un-Oatmeal Cookie Recipe

Ingredients:
- 1 cup pitted medjool dates
- ½ cup pecans
- 3 tbsp coconut oil
- 2 eggs
- ¾ cup coconut flour
- ½ cup golden flax meal
- ¼ cup shredded, unsweetened coconut
- ½ cup raisins
- 1 tspn cinnamon
- 1 tsp vanilla
- Dash of salt

Directions: Preheat oven to 350°F. In the food processor, pulse the dates and pecans until they are coarsely chopped. Add coconut oil and eggs. Pulse until blended. Add coconut flour, golden flax meal, cinnamon, vanilla, and salt.

Pulse until mixed and a dough forms.

Remove dough to a large bowl. Add raisins and shredded coconut. Mix well with a large wooden spoon.

Line a cookie sheet with parchment paper. Drop dough by the tablespoon-full onto the paper. Bake until the cookies set and begin to turn brown, about 12 – 15 minutes. Remove from oven and cool on pan or baking rack.

Serving size: 1 cookie   Yields: 15 servings
Prep time: 10 min   Bake time: 15 minutes   Total time: 25 min

*If you have decided not to use flax in your Paleo plan, you can substitute almond flour for the golden flax meal.

CONDIMENTS

- Catsup -

- Honey Mustard Dip -

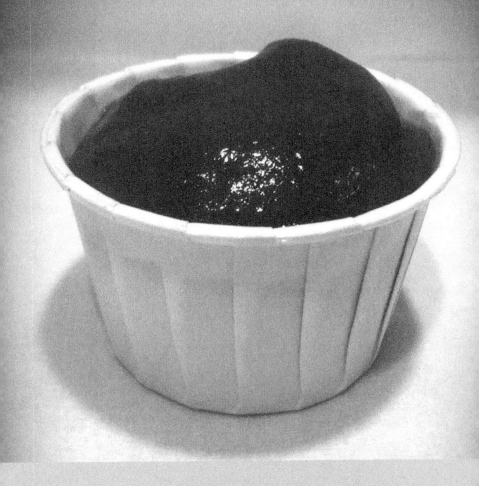

Catsup

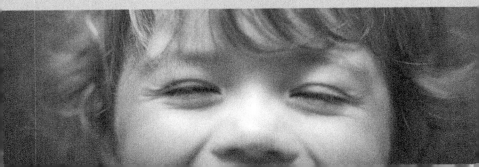

CATSUP

My daughter eats catsup with everything... eggs, fries, sausage. Sometimes I'll even see her dipping her carrot sticks in it! But regular catsup is off-limits on the Paleo diet, so I had to come up with an alternative that was going to please my catsup-connosseur's picky palate. This one not only makes her happy, it's easy to prepare... so it makes me happy, too.

Catsup Recipe

Ingredients:
- 5 oz (two cartons) "just prunes" organic baby food
- 5 oz tomato paste
- 1 ½ tsp lemon juice
- 1 ½ tsp raw honey, softened
- ¼ tsp ground mustard powder
- ¼ tsp sea salt

Directions: In a medium sized bowl, whisk all ingredients together until smooth. Store in an airtight container in the refrigerator up to two weeks.

*This is a basic recipe. You can give it your own flare by adding garlic powder, cumin, nutmeg, cinnamon, red chili powder, and more!

Serving size: 1 tbsp   Yields: 10 servings
Prep time: 3 min   Cook time: 0
Total: 3 minutes

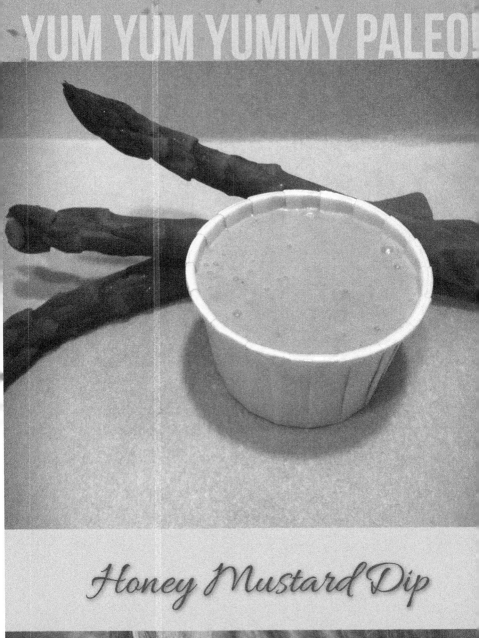

Honey Mustard Dip

HONEY MUSTARD DIP

Nothing goes better with a chicken strip than a little cup of honey mustard. Now, my daughter would argue that catsup is best until the cows (or chickens) come home, but that's why we've included both of these condiments... choice is key in making this diet plan work for everyone! You can also use this recipe as a dressing for salads or as a veggie dip.

Honey Mustard Dip Recipe

Ingredients:
- 3 tbsp raw honey
- 1 ½ tsp ground mustard
- 2 tsp lemon juice
- 3 tbsp olive oil
- ¼ tsp salt
- Pepper to taste

Directions: In a food processor, blend raw honey, lemon juice, and mustard powder until well blended. While blade is running, slowly drizzle in the olive oil until fully blended. Add salt and pepper to taste and pule one time to mix. Store in a container in the fridge up to two weeks.

Serving size: 1 teaspoon   Yields: 16 teaspoons
Prep time: 5 min   Cook time: 0
Total: 5 min

YUM YUM YUMMY SNACKS!

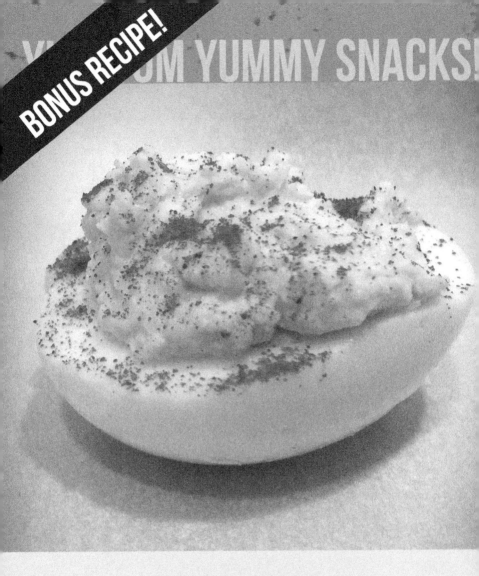

Deviled Eggs

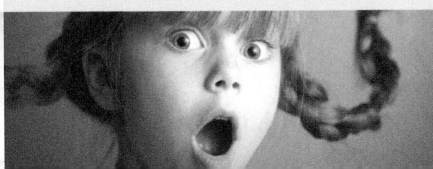

DEVILED EGGS
(BONUS RECIPE FROM *PALEO KID SNACKS*)

Eggs are a great source of protein on the Paleo diet. I like to boil a dozen at the beginning of the week just to have on hand for quick snacks. But when you don't want just a plain old egg, you can create a delicious appetizer in just a few quick steps.

Deviled Eggs Recipe

Ingredients:
- 2 boiled eggs
- 3 tsp Paleo mayonnaise (recipe from *Paleo Kid Snacks*)
- Dash paprika (optional)

Directions: Slice the boiled eggs in half lengthwise. Gently remove the yolk into a medium sized bowl. To the yolk, add 3 teaspoons mayonnaise. Mash with a fork, and then whip until the mixture is smooth. Scoop about 1 teaspoon of mixture back into each egg-white half. Sprinkle with paprika.

Serving size: 2 halves   Yields: 2 servings
Prep time: 5 minutes (from pre-boiled eggs)   Cook time: 0
Total time: 5 minutes

ABOUT THE AUTHOR

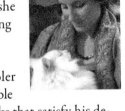

Kate Evans Scott is a stay-at-home mom to a preschooler and a toddler. In her former life she worked in graphic design and publishing which she now draws from to create inspiring books for young children and parents.

Her passion for writing began with her preschooler who is an encyclopedia of all things animal, vegetable and mineral. With a deep interest to create books that satisfy his desire to learn, and his love of food, Kids Love Press was born.

MORE BOOKS FROM KIDS LOVE PRESS:

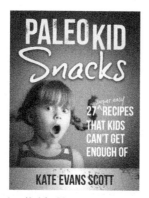

Available Now on Amazon

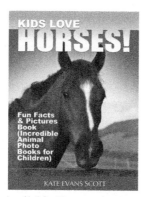

Available Now on Amazon

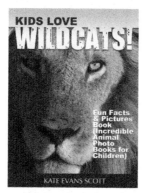

Available Now on Amazon

NOTES

NOTES

CPSIA information can be obtained at www.ICGtesting.com
Printed in the USA
LVOW04s1446151015

458413LV00014B/729/P